DETERMINING MARIJUANA USE IN THE AGE OF LEGALIZATION

G. Scott Graham

Independently Published

Copyright © 2019 G. Scott Graham

All rights reserved

The characters and events portrayed in this book are fictitious. Any similarity to real persons, living or dead, is coincidental and not intended by the author.

No part of this book may be reproduced, or stored in a retrieval system, or transmitted in any form or by any means, electronic, mechanical, photocopying, recording, or otherwise, without express written permission of the publisher.

ISBN-13: 9798746503084

Library of Congress Control Number: 2018675309
Printed in the United States of America

"Why do I do it? Because I enjoy its effects. You know, I - why does anybody use any mind-altering substance, you know, because they like the way it makes them feel."

MARK STEPNOSKI

CONTENTS

Title Page	
Copyright	
Epigraph	
Forward	1
Preface	7
About Me	9
About This Book	10
Marijuana from a Social Perspective	11
Snake Oil Marketing	13
Propaganda fueled by Anecdotal Hype	15
I. Introduction	17
The Changing Face of Marijuana Consumption, Myths and Use	19
Today's Legal Marijuana	22
Treatment Concerns: The Potency of Alcohol and Determining Consumption	23
Treatment Concerns: The Potency of Marijuana and Determining Consumption	25
Why clinicians need to be concerned with this	27
II. Developing a comparable measurement for THC	31
Overview	33

Percentage in Flowers	34
Milligrams (mg) in Everything Else	35
The relationship between percent THC and mg: doing marijuana math	36
Joint - a common but rough measurement	38
III. Two issues when assessing smoking marijuana flower	41
Overview	43
Sharing	44
Efficiency	45
IV. Converting Flower from percent to milligrams per serving – Summary	47
Four Step Summary	48
Converting Flower from percent to milligrams per serving - Example	49
V. Marijuana Products	51
Overview / General Considerations	53
Additional Considerations with Vaping	54
VI. Two Potential Screening Topics	55
Overview	57
Have you ever over-consumed an edible?	58
Microdosing	60
VII. The Future	63
Appendix	69
Counselor Bias Toward the Legal Use of Marijuana	71
Glossary of Terms Used in this Text plus!	81
Cannabis Consumption Calculator (CCC)	85
Hookles	89
Bibliography: A Curated Reading List	93
End Notes	109

List of Contributors	111
About Scott Graham	113
Other Books by Scott Graham	115
Contact Scott Graham	117

FORWARD

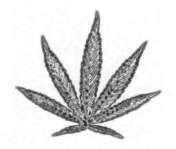

G. SCOTT GRAHAM

"If you substitute marijuana for tobacco and alcohol, you'll add eight to 24 years to your life."

JACK HERER

Scott Graham has had some interesting careers in his life! I first met him in the early 90's when we worked at an adventure-based adolescent treatment facility in New Hampshire (where he once had a client carry a toilet plunger all day for some kind of Reality Therapy session). Several years later, we both worked for the State of Vermont where he provided treatment to offenders with substance use disorders, and I worked down the hall in prevention trying to keep his caseload down. Scott now works as a certified life coach, EMT, author and hosts international volunteers who help him with the myriad of rescue animals living on his farm (including llamas, bunny rabbits and pot-bellied pigs). Currently, Scott and I cross paths together, literally, while hiking in the White Mountains with our dogs. We have many animated conversations about politics, culture and the current state of affairs. And of course, we talk about our jobs and how the legalized adult use of marijuana is changing the landscape in our work in prevention and treatment.

One way the landscape is shifting is how the cannabis industry attempts to normalize marijuana by adopting medical terminology in order to market it as a safe and healthy "product," but we all know cannabis/marijuana IS a drug. And like any other drug, whether used medically or recreationally, it can be misused and abused. Recreational adult-use marijuana is now sold in "dispensaries" and sellers tell you what "dosage" you should buy. But how does one really measure the dosage of THC or ascertain if use is excessive? What is the amount we should tell a client to cut back on if there are problems and how is this level determined? We can ask questions found in the DSM 5 or CUDIT-R, but unlike alcohol, there is no current way to measure how much consumption is occurring or what a moderate, socially responsible, adult level of use might look like. Knowing more about dosage and potency of THC can help clinicians better assess their clients and this book will help to set a course to do just that.

Case in point, we all have that friend, family member or client who uses or misuses alcohol to self-medicate. You know, that person with social anxiety who drinks at a party to get some "liquid courage" so they feel more confident, become more talkative, and experience less anxiety? These people still have anxiety, but the drug alcohol helps them temporarily relieve this emotion. Despite this self medicating, one would never call a local bar an alcohol "dispensary." They would never ask a bartender for medical advice on what "dosage" of alcohol or level of intoxication they need to achieve to be less anxious or to sleep better, right? (We all know that alcohol depletes melatonin anyway, so it really is not a good sleep aide on any account). Alcohol is a drug that is used socially and the standard measurements that have been developed to help what excessive use looks like are critical to interventions and treatment.

But what happens when the drug of choice is marijuana?

In the age of marijuana legalization and commercialization, this book is a timely primer for all Counselors, Addiction workers, Preventionists and others working in the field. As a Certified

Prevention Consultant in Vermont for 27 years, I know all too well that we cannot ignore that marijuana is not necessarily the "harmless" drug or a cure-all that many claim. And while we are waiting for deeper and more statistically valid research to truly ascertain the medicinal qualities of marijuana, or know people who use marijuana without issues, there are still those people who are harmed by the use/misuse of marijuana and or its potential side effects, including addiction. Having a method to better quantify the frequency of use and level of THC exposure, can help therapists, counselors, friends and loved ones better serve those who seek treatment or are concerned about their level of marijuana use.

Robin Rieske, MS, Certified Prevention Consultant
Co-Author - Substance Abuse Certification Training Manual ,
DCLAS, 2006-2014
Brattleboro, VT

PREFACE

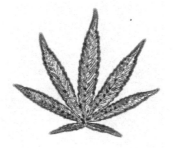

"If the whole world smoked a joint at the same time, there would be world peace for at least two hours."

UNKNOWN

ABOUT ME

I have worked in the addictions field since 1987. I am a Licensed Alcohol and Drug Abuse Counselor.

I have worked as a Prevention Specialist with inner city youth in Tampa Florida and a survival guide with teen age addicts in the Oregon wilderness and an outpatient counselor / clinical supervisor / program director in a 9-month statewide treatment program for Vermont Department of Corrections.

I have taught substance abuse courses at the college level.

I co-own a bar. We are the third largest seller of Jack Daniels in the entire state of New Hampshire.

One of my hobbies is making Mead (honey wine).

I support marijuana legalization.

My favorite alcohol product is Guinness (on tap, mind you, from a nitrogen tap).

My favorite marijuana product is infused tincture (at 1 mg / drop).

For fun, I would choose marijuana over alcohol any day of the week.

ABOUT THIS BOOK

This book is about marijuana. Legal marijuana. It's about the future of legal marijuana.

So many aspects described in this book may not apply to your specific geographic area depending on the legal status of marijuana where you work and live.

If you are in an area where marijuana is illegal (including the medical use of marijuana), consider yourself lucky. Lucky to be able to tap into the experience of other people who have forged ahead with legalization. Lucky to learn from their wise decisions. Lucky to learn from their mistakes.

MARIJUANA FROM A SOCIAL PERSPECTIVE

The framing of drugs, socially, has an interesting impact. Consider the drug alcohol. People drink alcohol to get a buzz (recreational use) but at the same time there is a big social aspect. Somebody wins something and they get champagne shaken and sprayed on them. We ring in the new year with champagne. The framing of marijuana is from a medical perspective. Even though smoking a joint couldn't be more social!
Just like you can't picture someone winning a race and having a bunch of people blow marijuana smoke on them as a sign of congratulations. You wouldn't picture someone drinking from a glass a wine and passing it around for all their friends to have a sip!

In their push for legalization, the marijuana industry frames marijuana as a curative for not only physical conditions but mental and emotional conditions. Medical relief first, recreation second.

This is important for health professionals because one of the markers used to identify the progress of addictive behaviors is the shift from recreational use to coping. (Occasional Relief Drinking is one marker ad is the onset of Constant Relief Drinking). So what happens is the initial use is from the perspective of relief? And how do we manage it when an employee demands to come to work high because they are anxious and if we don't allow them to drive a bus load of school kids when they are stoned we are discriminating against them?

You might laugh at this and think that there is no way that a situation like this could occur. But a few years ago, people would have been just as incredulous at the thought of someone bringing an emotional support peacock on a plane flight sitting on its own seat for free because it is a service animal yet that is exactly the situation we got into. A whole market of fake certifications including certificates, official looking IDs and fake vests to put on your pet in order to take them places where pets are not allowed have emerged because public policy makers were sloppy in defining what a service animal was and human service professionals for one reason or another never took a stand on it.

In this emerging world, public policy makers must navigate between two competing commentaries:

1. the pro marijuana people and the
2. anti-marijuana people.

Writing a book about a charged issue like marijuana would fail if it did not acknowledge these two opposing perspectives and their impact on public health information and legalization process. In this book, I strive to present these two perspectives objectively and directly – educating you, the reader, to the biases inherent in each perspective.

SNAKE OIL MARKETING

First the Pro-marijuana people. They won't be happy until you can go down to the Quick Mart and choose between the no-alcohol THC "infused" beer and the alcoholic beers and wines that are displayed for you to purchase. These people have leveraged the magical medicinal use of cannabinoids (there are over one hundred of them) including THC and CDB to cure everything from migraines to athlete's foot. It is snake oil marketing designed to get you to buy into the mysterious powers of marijuana and get it into your home. One friend defended their snake oil habit saying, "one 5 mg watermelon lozenge and I sleep so much better at night." Well a snifter of brandy will do the same thing yet we would be concerned about someone who habitually drank alcohol before bed each night in addition to other use of alcohol. Similarly, another friend defended their use of "one drop of indica tincture a couple of times a day because it helped her feel less anxious in her work." Well if she was drinking a margarita a couple of times a day to feel less anxious in her work, we might be concerned.

Medical mumbo jumbo and symptom justification. I am not buying it. Consider the term dispensary. This is a loaded term designed to *frame* the conversation around marijuana from a medical perspective.

But these dispensaries ARE NOT pharmacies. Think of the last time you went to get a PRESCIRPTION MEDICINE. Not only is a pharmacist available to talk to you about the medicine, you actually have to sign something declining a consult with the pharmacist. AND you get sheets and sheets of paper stuffed in your shopping bag along with the medication about side effects, conditions for not using etc. Right? Not so when you go to the cannabis dispensary to pick up your dose. In fact, a study by doctors at Denver Health and the University Of Colorado School Of Medicine in 2018 reported that the majority of the 280 marijuana stores in Colorado suggested cannabis for pregnancy-related nausea (morning sickness) while health experts, regulatory officials and even industry advocates warned against that! [i]

For that reason, you will see me see the term *marijuana store* instead of *dispensary* here. You will also see the term *serving* instead of *dose*. There certainly are medical uses for marijuana, my spouse who has Lyme's disease claims decreased pain since taking 20 mg CBD twice each day and taking a couple of hits from a marijuana vape pen at night.

You will also see the concept of recreational use highlighted and referenced repeatedly. One of the pieces of feedback I received in the process of writing this book was a suggestion to not use the term recreational use. "Legal consumption" I was told, "C'mon. People get high for one reason. And that is the same reason for alcohol: the effects." To put it simply, marijuana is fun.

PROPAGANDA FUELED BY ANECDOTAL HYPE

Now on to the anti-marijuana people. These people won't be happy until there is complete prohibition again. They flood the discussion with emotional charged anecdotal stories. like Newsweek story of the "Man Who Ate Marijuana Lollipop Had Heart Attack Caused by 'Fearful Hallucinations'." [ii]

Stories likes this becomes a mantra of health professionals warning you to stay away from edibles because you could have a heart attack and die or more evidence that marijuana is dangerous and should be avoided if you want to live a long and healthy life.

Yet you don't see these health professionals warning about the dangers of drinking water. Like the CBS story of the teen who died from drinking too much water during football practice.[iii]

You don't see these health professionals running around warning you to stay away from water because you could die from drinking it claiming it as evidence that water is dangerous and should be avoided if you want to live a long and healthy life. Can you end up in the Emergency Room from consuming too much marijuana edibles? Sure. Could you end up in the Emergency Room from drinking too much water. Absolutely. But people don't go around with a personal bias against water. They do go around with a personal bias against marijuana.

Trouble
I am troubled by the helter skelter avalanche of marijuana products brought on my legalization and foresee some big trouble down the road unless health professionals and public policy makers create a clear easy-to-understand method of determining a "serving" of marijuana.

Big trouble.

That's why I wrote this book.

What we really need is clear labeling and consumption guidelines. This won't happen until there is a standard for measuring and communicating the amount of THC across products. I hope that this book helps bridge the gap by outlining a formula to help counselors determine the consumption level across various products.

G. Scott Graham
March, 2019

I. INTRODUCTION

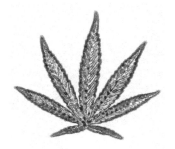

"It's no wonder that truth is stranger than fiction. Fiction has to make sense."

MARK TWAIN

THE CHANGING FACE OF MARIJUANA CONSUMPTION, MYTHS AND USE

There was a time when you purchased a bag of pot from a friend or neighbor or connection and had no idea of what you were getting. Today you can get marijuana legally in many forms flowers to concentrates to edibles to infusions to pre-measured vape pens to transdermal patches to suppositories. The days of dubious products from illegal markets are disappearing. With lab quality marijuana, driven by a medical-use focus secondary to a recreational focus, dosing is becoming more measurable and understandable.

The Rhetoric of Health Professionals
Health professionals warned of the dangers of purchasing marijuana, emphasizing that you didn't know what you were buying. Even recently, at a training for EMS (Emergency Medical Services) providers in Vermont that I trained, one presenter even claimed that marijuana was being mixed with "bath salts".

Now there was a case in 2013 described in "Bath Salts-Induced Psychosis: A Case Report" in Innovations in Clinical Neuroscience that described a 15 year old boy who became agitated and psychotic after reportedly smoking marijuana laced with bath salts.[iv] An article in Fire Engineering also identified consumption o f bath salts to get high as an "emerging threat."[v]

This issue (and other scare tactics like it) are not at all applicable to legal marijuana purchased from a legal marijuana store today. The legal marijuana industry is heavily regulated and monitored with multiple safe guards built in

Another scare tactic you may have heard of its potency. Many health professionals today emphasize the potency shift from the 1960s to today. Statements like this, which ignore some of the flaws in the studies that generated these conclusions[vi], might only be helpful to a 50 year old who smoked pot in the 60s and now expects the SAME EFFECT from the SAME AMOUNT of marijuana smoked. The issue is not potency.

The issue is that we have no common framework to determine potency across marijuana products like we do with alcohol.

(Actually consumers high potency is good news! This information is not considered a warning but a testament that products are of good quality).

The Rhetoric from the ~~Marijuana~~ Cannabis Industry

At the same time that some health professionals are trying to scare you into abstinence, the marijuana industry – I mean, er, "cannabis" industry is working hard to change the image of the pot user so that consumption of marijuana is not only legal but normal – a strategy driven by their bottom line, money.

The marijuana industry – eyes glazed with the promise of big profits -- are working hard to change the image of pot from something purchased in back alleys to something you can consume in polite society, starting with the words you use to describe everything from consumption to the industry itself.

You will never hear these people say "marijuana". They claim that the term marijuana is racist (fake news). We should use the term "cannabis" they say.

You will also hear the terms "dose" (how much you consume at any one time), "dispensary" (where you go these days to buy pot), and "psychoactive effects" (getting high). Their agenda is to make marijuana acceptable and is grounded in *medical* lingo because the legalization process is typically medical marijuana first, recreational use second.

TODAY'S LEGAL MARIJUANA

Today's marijuana products are clearly labeled so that consumers know what they are buying.
This is driven primarily from an economic perspective and an effort to make sure consumers aren't getting ripped off by various marijuana producers. It is also driven by a legal perspective. In many places there is a legal limit to how much marijuana an individual can possess, and the marijuana sellers don't want those consumers who purchase an assortment of marijuana products are not subject to arrest on their way home.

Unfortunately, this detailed measuring and labeling is not done from a public health perspective. As the legalization movement continues to unfold, public health professionals must engage and influence the discussion so that at some point in the future normal use can be *easily* differentiated from use that may be problematic or even dangerous. Until that time, counselors and other public health professionals will need to be mathematicians in order to have a quantity and potency that is comparable across the range of marijuana products (including marijuana flower) that is available.

TREATMENT CONCERNS: THE POTENCY OF ALCOHOL AND DETERMINING CONSUMPTION

Three clients come into your office. In a routine inquiry you ask each about their alcohol consumption. The first client reports drinking a bottle of wine each night as she prepares dinner. The second client reports that he drinks an 18-pack of beer over the course of a week with the majority of it on the weekend. The third reports that she has two martinis after she gets home from work on weekdays.

Most health professionals would have little difficulty determining alcohol use of concern – alcohol use that would prompt for further assessment. Thanks to guidelines provided by the US Government: "moderate alcohol consumption is defined as having up to 1 drink per day for women and up to 2 drinks per day for men. This definition refers to the amount consumed on any single day and is not intended as an average over several days." (https://health.gov/dietaryguidelines/2015/guidelines/appendix-9/). Excessive (or heavy) drinking is defined as consuming 15 drinks or more per week for me and consuming 8 drinks or more per week for women (https://www.cdc.gov/alcohol/faqs.htm).

Furthermore, thanks to the U.S. Departments of Health and Human Services and Agriculture, we know that a drink of alcohol is "12 oz. of regular beer, 5 oz. of wine, and 1.5 oz. of 80-proof distilled spirits."

Finally thanks to the concept of proof -- a term that dates back over 400 years to England where alcohol was taxed based on the amount of ethanol in it (proof = percentage ethanol times two) (https://en.wikipedia.org/wiki/Alcohol_proof), we know that 1.5 ounces of 80 proof alcohol contains twice as much ethanol as 1.5 ounces of 40 proof alcohol.

While it is true that excessive alcohol consumption does not mean severe alcohol use disorder (most people who drink heavily do not meet the clinical diagnostic criteria for severe alcohol use disorder BUT at the same time most people who meet the clinical diagnostic criteria for alcohol use disorder do drink heavily), the guideline provides a starting point for discussion around alcohol use and health while also providing a data point for assessing tolerance increase (which is a diagnostic criteria for alcohol use disorder).

TREATMENT CONCERNS: THE POTENCY OF MARIJUANA AND DETERMINING CONSUMPTION

The next day, three more clients come into your office. In a routine inquiry you ask each about their marijuana consumption. The first client reports sharing half a joint of "walker kush" each night with her husband before dinner. The second client reports that he uses a 200mg vape pen every hour throughout the day -- sometimes more -- and inhales for about "2-seconds". The third reports that she has two "blue-raspberry" marijuana cocktails (alcohol-free) after she gets home from work made with "10 drops of indicia tincture, organic blueberry juice, frozen wild raspberries and 1/4 teaspoon of wheat grass."

Most health professional would struggle with determining marijuana use of concern. In fact most health professionals would be completely bewildered in comparing these different products and methods of consumption. There are no such guidelines for marijuana consumption like there are for alcohol.

WHY CLINICIANS NEED TO BE CONCERNED WITH THIS

You might be asking why we need a system of measurement for marijuana consumption like we do for alcohol. After all the DSM5 is clear in outlining substance use disorders: 11 criteria to evaluate and "mild" "moderate" and "severe" specifiers depending on the number of criteria present. Cannabis Use Disorder Criteria (DSM 5):

1. Taking more than was intended
2. Difficulty controlling or cutting down
3. Spending a lot of time on use
4. Craving
5. Problems at work, school, and home as a result of use
6. Continuing to use despite social or relationship problems
7. Giving up or reducing other activities in favor of cannabis
8. Taking cannabis in high-risk situations
9. Continuing to use cannabis despite physical or psychological problems
10. Tolerance to cannabis

11. Withdrawal when discontinuing cannabis

Now when someone strolls into an office we just don't open the DSM to page one and go through diagnosis after diagnosis, criteria after criteria, and question after question to assess and identify problematic areas for treatment. We listen to the client's history and symptoms to discern whether we need to explore deeper using assessment instruments and the DSM.

Illicit use is often a cue to look deeper for public health professionals who are screening then assessing for addiction. For example, consider a client who comes into your office and discloses IV heroin use, you probably deduce that this client may have an opiod use disorder and flip open your DSM to the appropriate page and ask some questions.

With legal substances, your approach is probably different. A client who comes to your office and says they drink alcohol does not prompt you to open the DSM and ask if their drinking has created social or relationship problems. You probably ask one question to determine your next step: "How much?" Their answer to this question prompts to either move on or explore more deeply the substance being discussed.

How can you have a conversation about marijuana use and health when you have no idea of the amount of THC being consumed?

Further consider this: If we can't quantify THC consumption then how can we determine – or help a client determine -- tolerance?

According to the 2015 National Survey on Drug Use and Health (NSDUH), 56.0 percent of people ages 18 or older reported that they drank during the past month. What happens when marijuana use reaches that percentage – when over half the people you know report that they consumed THC in one form or the other during the past month?

Health professionals need to be able to quantify "how much."

The Myth of "Personalized Prescription"

The marijuana industry would like to defocus you by claiming that things like dose (aka serving size) are an individual matter and totally dependent on the individual.

This is just silly. It is not an excuse to calculate precise measurements for consumption.

Certainly people metabolize THC at different rates. People also metabolize ethanol at different rates AND its impact is also dependent on tolerance. That "fact" hasn't stopped health professionals and government leaders from developing a comparative measurement across alcohol products and identifying legal limits for driving, and recommendations for daily / weekly consumption habits.

This whole "it's personal" thing by the marijuana industry is just rhetoric designed to derail efforts for regulation. Don't buy it!

II. DEVELOPING A COMPARABLE MEASUREMENT FOR THC

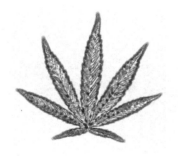

"Science cannot progress without reliable and accurate measurement of what it is you are trying to study. The key is measurement, simple as that."

ROBERT D. HARE

OVERVIEW

THC is the psychoactive substance in marijuana, like ethanol is the intoxicating substance in alcohol. As stated in the introduction, primarily for economic, regulatory and legal reasons, there have been steps taken to standardized (and even insure) the potency of the different marijuana-based products (note the marijuana study for Colorado). In order to determine use, we must understand potency across products.

PERCENTAGE IN FLOWERS

THC is measured in percent in marijuana flowers when you purchase them at a dispensary including flower products like pre-rolled joints. Clients know what they are buying today. Simply ask about the percentage THC in the flower. Informed users will know -- so don't take "I don't know" for an answer.

Someone buys flower that is listed at 25% THC and rolls a joint, holds it in their hand and shows it to you. At the risk of oversimplifying, ¼ of what you see is THC and ¾ of what you see is other stuff. Now you may think that you can just cut off a quarter of the joint and have just the THC part and throw the rest away. But that is not true: THC is distributed throughout the whole flower at 25%.

MILLIGRAMS (MG) IN EVERYTHING ELSE

Milligrams (or mg) is the other number you'll see at marijuana stores (aka "dispensaries"). Whether on pre-measured vaporizer cartridges (often 200 mg, 300 mg, 500 mg or 1000 mg), edibles (100 mg dark chocolate bars, 5 mg gummies, 5 mg lozenges, etc), infused tinctures (typically 1 mg / drop), THC is identified by milligrams.

Someone buys an infused tincture and puts one drop in a spoon and holds it in their hand and shows it to you. You are told that that drop is 1 mg. That 1 mg is 100% THC. That one drop is 100% THC.

What we are talking about here is potency. The 25% THC in the flower example above describes the potency. When other products are created from marijuana that THC is turned into a concentrate and that concentrated is tested for potency. Then that concentrate is then mixed with other ingredients and a dosage calculated.

Those milligrams are 100% potent.

So you should be able to take 5 drops of tincture at 1 gram per drop and experience a similar effect as consuming a 5mg watermelon candy.

A milligram is a milligram is a milligram, in other words.

THE RELATIONSHIP BETWEEN PERCENT THC AND MG: DOING MARIJUANA MATH

So then the question is what do we do about marijuana in its flower form where THC is labeled as a percentage?

Just as there is a relationship between percent and proof ethanol for alcohol, there is a relationship between percent and milligrams THC for marijuana.

It does require some math but it is not too complicated. In fact all you have to do to convert THC percent to THC milligrams is move the decimal point. Buying one gram of flower that is 18.2% THC means you have 182 milligrams of THC in that flower.

The Math: 18.2% x 1 gram x 1000 milligrams/gram = 182 milligrams THC

It's not as easy when buying amounts different than a gram but the math is the same. If you purchase a pre-rolled joint that is 0.75 grams and the THC is 18.2%, then...

The Math 18.2% x .75 gram x 1000 milligrams/gram = 136.5 milligrams THC

Since most everything sold at dispensaries describes THC in terms of milligrams with the notable exception of flower (which is sold by weight), it makes sense to think about THC consumption in terms of milligrams consumed and do the work to convert flowers smoked to milligrams consumed.

Now, I know what you are thinking: "How do we translate this to a discussion with a client and accurately assess how much THC they are consuming?" We need a common reference for flowers.

JOINT - A COMMON BUT ROUGH MEASUREMENT

Let's be clear. People don't think in terms of grams. So it could be challenging to figure out how much a person smoked of marijuana in its flower form.

A joint, however, presents a common – albeit admittedly still inaccurate measure and point of reference. It is like a dietician talking about sandwiches. To some, a sandwich is two pieces of bread and once piece of meat with some mustard. To others a sandwich is 10 pieces of meat, 5 pieces of cheese, four slices of tomato and mayonnaise. But most people can identify and agree upon a "typical" sandwich.

If you asked a person to estimate how many joints they smoked and they said "a half", you should be able to calculate grams THC consumed.

There are two assumptions you will make in your calculations:

1. We will make an assumption that the average joint = 1/2 gram
2. When someone does not know the percentage THC, assume 15%

With that conversion factor in mind a person who smokes half a joint has consumed 1/4 gram which you can plug into the equation above to determine milligrams THC consumed.

The Math for the "I don't know percent THC" 15% x .25 gram x 1000 milligrams/gram = 37.5 milligrams THC

III. TWO ISSUES WHEN ASSESSING SMOKING MARIJUANA FLOWER

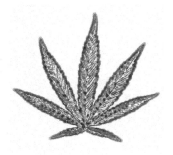

"It is the mark of an educated man to look for precision in each class of things just so far as the nature of the subject admits"

ARISTOTLE

OVERVIEW

There are two other factors when converting THC percentage in flower to milligrams per serving: sharing and efficiency. Unique to marijuana use is the culture of sharing: people do not typically smoke marijuana flower alone. And the absorption of THC through the lungs is impacted by the act of smoking itself: so much of the THC literally goes "up in smoke."

SHARING

Products created with THC concentrates are not shared -- at least not in the usual way that smoking flower has been shared. Someone might offer 10 mg piece of their dark chocolate bar or a 5mg watermelon gummy, but they aren't going to take a 5mg lozenge, take a lick pass it to their friend who takes a lick who then passes it to another who takes a lick as it moves around the room back to the original "licker." In other words, because marijuana products are discrete in terms of both packaging and mg THC it is much easier to determine mg THC consumed. Marijuana in its flower form is often shared. Traditionally you don't see 5 people in a room each smoking their own joint. There is usually one joint that is passed around from person to person.

Because of this, it is important to consider in our percent THC to mg calculation if the marijuana was shared and if so with how many other people. Note that the number should be the total number of people sharing including the person reporting. So 1 person sharing with 3 others who smoked an entire joint means that person has consumed 1/4 of a joint and not an entire joint. We are of course making an assumption that everyone equally consumed that joint. It is our best calculation given how flower is typically smoked.

EFFICIENCY

Smoking marijuana in its flower form is the most inefficient method for consuming marijuana. Some calculate that 70% of the THC is lost in the process of smoking. This does not happen with products created from marijuana. Those products are at 100% potency and deliver 100% potency when consumed. Their potency is measured after the THC is released via decarbing and then standardized when packaging.

In order to get an accurate measure of THC consumed from smoking marijuana in its flower form, we need to consider potency lost from smoking in our calculations:

> A 50% loss calculation is easy and probably acceptable. In other words you will be dividing your final number by two to account for sidestream loss while smoking.

IV. CONVERTING FLOWER FROM PERCENT TO MILLIGRAMS PER SERVING – SUMMARY

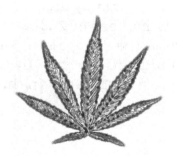

FOUR STEP SUMMARY

1. Convert percentage to milligrams per gram. If the client does not know the percent, assume 15% THC.
2. Calculate amount consumed using a joint as a measurement
    a. how many joints smoked divided by
    b. the number of people smoking divided by
    c. two (50% THC lost to the sidestream) yields
    d. the amount smoked in joints
3. Convert joint to gram by dividing the amount smoked in joints (the number in 2 above) by two (remember that we assume the average joint = 1/2 gram)
4. Multiply milligrams per gram by the amount of grams smoked to yield the THC serving in milligrams.

CONVERTING FLOWER FROM PERCENT TO MILLIGRAMS PER SERVING - EXAMPLE

Fred reports smoking "Sweet Tooth" with 3 friends. "Sweet Tooth" is sold at 27.4% THC. Fred states that they smoked the entire joint.

Here are the answers following the steps above:

1. 274 milligrams THC per gram
2. 1/8 joint smoked (1 divided by 4 multiplied by 50% OR, easier, 1 divided by 4 divided by 2)
    a. 1 joint, *shared by*
    b. 4 people
    c. 50% *lost to the sidestream*
3. 1/16 gram
4. 274 x (1/16) = 17.12 milligrams THC smoked.

Because this is a calculation, although relatively simple, it is recommended that public health professionals show their math (just like you did in school) so that the conversion from percent to milligrams is clear.

V. MARIJUANA PRODUCTS

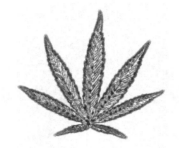

"From sleep aids to beverages, the future of cannabis is in products"

BRUCE LINTON, CANOPY CEO

OVERVIEW / GENERAL CONSIDERATIONS

Marijuana products are clearly labeled in mg so there is no math conversion. However, there are a few things to consider when asking about pre-packaged products. The math you need to do simply is to determine the servings in a specific product and how much is consumed. The dispensaries have worked to make this easy for consumers so clinicians should have no trouble. For example a chocolate bar containing 50 mg THC is scored to be broken into 10 pieces which means 5 mg (50 divided by 10) per piece. The same is true for vape pens (which shut off after a specific time period meaning a specific does) and infused oils or tinctures.

ADDITIONAL CONSIDERATIONS WITH VAPING

Full or partial inhale?

Most vape pens shut off after a period of inhalation. That might range from 5-7 seconds depending on the vape pen. A full inhalation delivers a full serving as labeled on the box. For example, a client may have a 200 mg vial that is essentially 100 2 mg servings (I know servings is probably a bad term to use but it is a familiar term). The client pen delivers that 2 mg serving over a 6-second inhale. So if a client inhales for 3 seconds instead of 6 they are getting half of a serving or 1 mg. Another client swaps out that vial for a vial that contains 1000 mg (one hundred, 10-mg servings). If that client also does one 3-second inhale, the client consumed 5 mg.

VI. TWO POTENTIAL SCREENING TOPICS

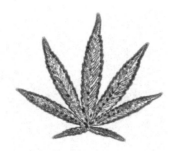

"The world is full of obvious things which nobody by any chance ever observes."

ARTHUR CONAN DOYLE

OVERVIEW

With alcohol, health professionals have an arsenal of screening tools at their disposal to help identify individuals in need of further assessment. There are two behavior areas that health professionals should consider when screening a client to determine if a more in-depth exploration about marijuana use is in order:
1. over-consuming edibles
2. microdosing

HAVE YOU EVER OVER-CONSUMED AN EDIBLE?

We have seen this in the news a number of times and this is often offered as a warning by health professionals to show how dangerous edible marijuana products are. For example, John purchases a marijuana chocolate bar then eats the whole thing. He ends up in the Emergency Room because he is anxious, hallucinating and freaking everybody out. But public health professionals should keep in mind that there is a diagnostic perspective to this behavior. An experienced user presenting the same behaviors is quite another matter. Consider the mental volition of the experienced user who tells you they have over-consumed edibles on more than one occasion. What is going on there? What is their mental volition? This behavior may be an indication of "chasing the high." The alcohol-use equivalent might be a person doing 3 shots of tequila one right after another and then deciding to do 2 more shots and getting wasted. This experienced user (again I am emphasizing this is not a one-time accident) essentially gets impatient at the psychoactive results and then eats more edibles and then over-consumes.

Although there is no research yet about this behavior, it is one that public health professionals should be aware of because of its screening potential.

MICRODOSING

If there is one behavior that shows that the increase of THC potency over the past 30 years is a scare tactic myth, it is microdosing. Microdosing is an emerging behavior among some marijuana users and is only possible because of the specific measured delivery of THC in grams. Microdosing is possible because of products that contain a consistent, measured, small amount of THC in grams.

In microdosing, a person takes a small amount over a specific period of time all day long. Through microdosing, a person learns how their body responds to THC (the psychoactive effects) and then takes small servings to maintain that psychoactive effect they desire all day long. You might not even know a person who is microdosing is high (though they are experiencing psychoactive effects). With microdosing, gone are the days of smoking a joint and then being wasted on the couch for hours. With microdosing you can get a little high and still function quite normally all day long. This strategy certainly works great for pain management. Consider the person in discomfort who is able to alleviate that discomfort and still engage life – they are not a medicated zombie.

However, the recreational use of microdosing may have some diagnostic, screening value for the health professional. Let's explore this behavior around the use of alcohol. If a client came into your office and said that they drink alcohol all day long to help them get through the day, would this behavior raise some red flags for you? The client reports the they do not get drunk or pass out -- they basically have a cocktail every hour because it takes the edge off. All day long.

Compare that to a marijuana consumer who comes in and says they take four 1-mg drops in the morning with breakfast and then a drop an hour all day long to help him get through the day. He doesn't get wasted or pass out. It takes the edge off. All day long. Would this behavior raise some flags like the example of alcohol did above?

So while there is not a specific question about microdosing in the Cannabis Consumption Calculator™, exploring this area should probably be part of each public health professionals assessment process in areas where marijuana is legal, regulated and sold to adults.

VII. THE FUTURE

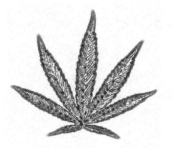

"Over the next 10 years, the legal cannabis industry is poised for explosive growth. Total spend on legal marijuana worldwide is expected to hit $57 billion by 2027. The recreational market is expected to cover 67 percent of this overall number, whereas medical marijuana is expected to comprise the remaining 33 percent."

ARCVIEW MARKET RESEARCH AND ITS RESEARCH PARTNER BDS ANALYTICS[VII]

The days of smoking a bowl or a joint are numbered.[viii] The writing is on the wall.

As marijuana use continues to be more acceptable and legal, and more and more people use it, marijuana products will soar in popularity and traditional flower will fade away from use from all but the romantics, purists and DIY-ers.

Consider the acceptance and growth of alcohol sales in the Unites States since the end of prohibition in 1933. Walk into any liquor store and you are bombarded with a myriad of alcohol choices, flavorings, proofs, concoctions and more. Today you can purchase grape-soda-flavored "malt beverages", in which one is hard pressed to discern any alcohol content. Our tastes have evolved from "bath tub gin".

Likewise the acceptance and growth of marijuana will produce a myriad of choices for consumers. And last on that list will be purchasing marijuana flower by the ounce or in pre-rolled joints. Marijuana products provide a clear choice when considering distinct packaging, controllable dosing and discrete consumption. Add to that the significant loss (up to 70%) of THC to the sidestream when smoked. And people will choose more efficient, surreptitious marijuana products. Consumers will always make the best buy for their money. In the world of marijuana that means processed, infused, products.

As the cannabis market develops and expands across the United States, more new consumers will become regular consumers. Cannabis businesses must adapt to this rapidly changing consumer landscape and stay ahead of developing trends to excel in tomorrow's industry.

From a business perspective:

"The most rapidly evolving product category is cannabis-infused edibles, which is projected to make up a $2.3-billion market in 2018 and to become a $5.3-billion market within the next five years (a 130-percent increase), according to data from cannabis market research firm Brightfield Group. Given those numbers, staying abreast of changing consumer preferences is probably a wise business decision." [ix]

It is noteworthy that this perspective is from business. Health professionals need to stay as equally abreast.

Now some may think that purchasing marijuana products for recreational use will be the domain of the affluent and people of less means will grow cannabis plants at home. Growing cannabis plants at home is a complex process with issues such as ph range, nutrient management, powdery mildew, bud rot, spider mites and aphids to deal with (just to name a few) in addition to managing harvest times and curing strategies. It is also an expensive process with thousands of dollars[x] for equipment outlays, including bulbs, fans, pots, watering systems and electricity. Home cultivation of cannabis plants will be similar like the home beer-making and home wine-making kits available on the market today – focused on the DIY-er who is interested home brewing as a hobby in and of itself and not as a way to get alcohol. Unlike the days before legalization, home cultivation of cannabis plants will not be the only means to get marijuana.

And it does appear that the current menu of products produced by the marijuana industry is just a start. Researchers are working on creating THC from synthetically-modified brewer's yeast[xi] and marijuana beer is now being sold (it's alcohol free by the way).[xii]

For policy makers, regulators and treatment providers the good news of this increased use of marijuana products instead of smoking marijuana flower, is that calculating use should become easier. At least health professionals won't have to convert from percentage to milligrams.

The bad news is that use (and misuse) becomes easier. Easier to manage. Easier to hide. Easier to abuse. All the more reason for public health professionals to advocate for a clear, understandable uniform label / measurement for THC.

APPENDIX

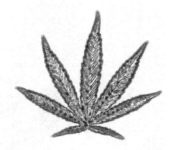

APPENDIX

COUNSELOR BIAS TOWARD THE LEGAL USE OF MARIJUANA

"Alcohol and marijuana, if used in moderation, plus loud, usually low-class music, make stress and boredom infinitely more bearable."

KURT VONNEGUT

Introduction

My thoughts are set down here in order to present the issue of my bias and to allow the reader to explore and consider his or her own personal situation through the framework of my experience. If you are a counselor, or even if you are not, change can be uncomfortable!

I must admit, I am feeling uneasy about the changes that appear to be coming. I'm OK with legalization of THC, which is long overdue. THC should be considered the same as alcohol, legal but not healthy for everybody, and certainly not to excess. And also considered the same as tobacco, which is legal but not healthy for anyone! And I'm not uneasy about the treatment perspective either. The abuse of any substance is a mental health issue. People who get into trouble with abusive or addictive behavior, whether it be drugs (including alcohol and tobacco, which are drugs), sex, gambling, etc, need support and guidance, and the counseling process is much the same.

And I do feel that the logistics will eventually be worked out, i.e. who can grow and how much, who can process, who can sell, gifting, labeling, taxes, and so on. Dealing with the change in social norms may be, in the long run, more of an issue.

Bias

To begin, let's be clear on the definition of the word "bias". Webster's Dictionary uses the words "prejudice" and "partiality", and the phrase "propensity of the mind", none of which sound very positive! Could these words apply to me??

Am I biased, or just concerned? I am uncomfortable with THC being used <u>recreationally,</u> even though I am okay with alcohol being used recreationally. I have no problem with folks enjoying a couple of drinks to socialize or relax. Therein lies the rub! (Bias does not always make sense!) If I feel okay with alcohol being used recreationally, will I adapt to the new social norms and get to the point where I feel comfortable with THC being used recreationally? What do YOU think of recreational THC and evolving social norms?

Recreational Use Versus Using To Cope

As a Licensed Alcohol and Drug Abuse Counselor, I know there is a big difference between using a substance recreationally and using it to cope. (The concept of occasional relief drinking as well as constant relief drinking are both markers in the Jellinek Curve developed by British psychiatrist Max Glatt and named after E.M. Jellinek, the American physiologist and researcher, on whose work this progression of addiction is based.) Alcohol can certainly be problematic if used as a coping mechanism. Should we use drugs when there are other ways to alter our moods or to cope with difficult feelings or situations? Talking through our issues with a friend or counselor, getting up and taking a walk or a run or a hike, taking an exercise class, volunteering, singing, laughing with friends, cooking a good meal, reading a good book or watching a favorite TV show (the list is endless) may be better choices. These same activities can help relieve stress, anxiety, and even pain, and create a sense of wellbeing. Is this a bias, or just sensible thinking?

Gaining Insight From History

When I analyze thoughts about THC being used recreationally, I realize that they sound like black and white thinking. How does anyone change black and white thinking?? Perhaps we begin by recognizing where it comes from, whether it affects one's behavior and judgment, and whether it is healthy for one to hang onto it.

As a I child, and for most of my adult life, I have lived in a rural area. Early on, which was a long time ago now, I was not aware of any illegal drug use in my community, and I believe there was very little or none. I remember an isolated instance when I was a teenager involving a friend's relative who was visiting from NYC and was brought along to a harmless teen party. He seemed obnoxious, laughing too loudly and generally out of control. I had no idea why, until someone whispered "marijuana". I did not see or hear about marijuana again in our area until men (boys really) started coming back from Vietnam, and so many of them were really messed up ...

Alcohol , on the other hand, had been around as far back as I can remember, of course. Every family had been affected by their own or someone else's alcohol use, and my family was no exception. There was an understood line between people who drank responsibly and people who were problem drinkers. Problem drinkers were thought of as weak, or bums, or people in the gutters. Illegal drugs were considered bad, and there was no "responsible use". (Most people now understand the nature of addiction, that people are victims of a disease, and modern research is teaching us it is a brain disease.)

I became certified as an addictions counselor in Vermont in 1998, almost 20 years before the date of this book's first publication. The trainings and education to become a counselor, and the continuing education courses and workshops since then to maintain my licensure as a Licensed Alcohol and Drug Counselor (LADC) were based on alcohol and illegal drugs. Marijuana had been illegal to purchase or possess seemingly forever, and illegal drug use of any kind was not okay from a treatment perspective. Treatment and recovery from alcohol and drug problems were generally based on abstinence. All the years of my practice as a counselor were based on this perspective.

Now, seemingly with the flipping of a switch, THC appears to be LEGALLY AND SOCIALLY accepted. I consider myself to be a pretty resilient person generally. However, this seems like it is a big change, and it appears to be happening very quickly. (In actuality, of course, it has been coming for many years.) Frankly, I am having some difficulty with it. Are you? If so, what are YOU going to do about it?

Clinical Issues

The two main issues that come to my mind for clinicians are: 1) How does this affect work with clients, and 2) How does this affect the clinician's family and social life, and perhaps one's own recovery?

If you are not a clinician, have you thought about how the legalization of THC could affect your personal, family, and social life?

The clinical issue is partly simple and partly complex. The simpler part is that if a client presents with issues around THC use, then as with any other substance, there is the usual counseling protocol of screening, intake, assessment, treatment planning or referral, etc.

The treatment plan for THC problems, just as for any other substance or behavioral problem, might include using less often or less amounts, or to use only on days or times that would not be as potentially problematic, or even to use a different form of THC. If a client is entering counseling due to a serious situation such as a criminal charge related to operating under the influence of THC, or the loss of employment or family due to using, then the plan could more likely be abstinence and identifying ways the client could meet his/her needs.

The more difficult part, for me and perhaps for you as well, might be to recognize and monitor any tension or bias in myself toward clients who use what was so long illegal. As always for counselors, the supervision piece is important, sharing treatment concerns with someone who is trusted and respected.

The next step might be to study how law and societal norms are changing, and the impact on our culture. This is an education piece. We can talk to others and attend workshops and trainings to understand the pluses and minuses of THC and what responsible use looks like. How do YOU feel, and what are YOU doing about it??

I have been attending new trainings and workshops on THC, so that as a counselor, I can provide up-to-date information and treatment on this mood altering drug. It used to be simple, with THC smoked and baked in brownies, but now there is so much more to know, including new information on the physiological and psychosocial aspects of this drug!! Even calling THC a "drug" begins to sound weird since we don't commonly call alcohol or tobacco drugs, even though they are! Must we all learn a new, common, language?

If you are a clinician who entered the treatment field due to your own experience battling addiction, does the legalization of THC and the change in societal norms affect your own lifelong recovery? Do you have a strong feelings about this? If so, what are you doing about it?

Family & Social Issues

Up until now, whether folks in my family or social network used or didn't use did not seem to matter much since if they did, they used in private, or at least not in my presence, and did not talk about it. Now, if people talk openly or use openly, how will I react?? Will I be surprised, repulsed, concerned?? Is it any of my business anyway?? How about you?

For those of us who choose not to use THC, will we feel pressure to use so we'll feel connected to a person or group?? What will we say if/when asked if we'd like a joint, puff, a brownie, whatever? Will it feel necessary to lie, to say: "Not today, thank you, I'm driving"? Or will we just gloss it over and say: "No thanks", and change the subject? Should we tell the complete truth--that we are non-users? (Is this what it feels like to "come out of the closet"?) Could we ask why THEY use? At a cocktail party, will we have to ask what is in the food or beverages (especially if we are in recovery)? Is this what feeling disconnected is like? Are we the only ones in the world not jumping on the bandwagon??

In our family lives, what if one's partner, children, or grandchildren begin to use, and perhaps use in our presence now that the law and societal norms have changed? How do we deal with that??

For now, maybe we try to relax and become observers of this legal and societal change. We can trust our skills at unconditional positive regard and respecting people's choices, whether they be our clients, friends, or family. We can like a person, but dislike their behavior. We'll figure this out....

A Note Of Caution For Counselors

If it seems like you have a bias, a word of caution for you and your peers: While you don't want to let your bias influence your treatment interactions with clients, at the same time, you don't want to swing in the other direction and just dismiss every conclusion you hold about marijuana. You also want to be vigilant that your peers don't dismiss YOU when discussing legal marijuana. ("Of COURSE, she is going to say that, she has issues with marijuana.") This is not only disrespectful and dismissive to you, but it is also not good critical clinical thinking.

Susan M. Williams, March 2019

GLOSSARY OF TERMS USED IN THIS TEXT PLUS!

A s I surveyed the legal marijuana industry and public health response to marijuana legalization, I came across some new terminology and some old terminology used with a new "spin" that I was not familiar with (at least in the context of the legal marijuana movement).

Cannabis – (a) "a genus of flowering plants in the family Cannabaceae. The number of species within the genus is disputed. Three species may be recognized: Cannabis sativa, Cannabis indica, and Cannabis ruderalis"[xiii]; (b) a marketing tactic by the marijuana industry framed as "politically correct".

Dispensary – (a) marijuana store; (b) a marketing tactic grounded in legal medical use which often precedes legal recreational use.

Dose – (a) how much THC you consume at one time; (b) can also be how much CBD you consume at one time; (c) defined as milligrams for marijuana products such as tinctures and edibles; (d) defined as one inhalation when smoking marijuana flower.

Flower – (a) a general term that refers to the smokeable part of a female cannabis plant. "Herb" is also used to refer to this but it is also a term used to refer to marijuana in general. (b) Flower seems to be the dominant term used in dispensaries. It is important to know because it refers to this specific form of marijuana as distinguished from other forms like tinctures, edibles.

Marijuana – (a) another name for cannabis; (b) a term you will hear labeled as "slang" and even "racist" (which it is not) by those in the legalization movement who want you to use the term cannabis instead.

Learn More Marijuana Terms

The Internet brings you a wealth or marijuana resources at your finger tips. Here are some suggested resources to get you going.

Colorado Pot Guide
The folks at Colorado Pot Guide have a great dictionary of marijuana terms. They claim they guide is "all you need to know about the world of marijuana from A-Z". There is a link for each term for more information and they also use it in a sentence so if you are worried about using a term incorrectly, you can check yourself.

https://www.coloradopotguide.com/marijuana-glossary/

Leafy
Leafy also has a dictionary -- it is not as long as the one above but all the terms are presented on one page

https://www.leafly.com/news/cannabis-101/glossary-of-cannabis-terms

Greencamp
Greencamp gives you a one page dictionary of 32 terms on one page aimed at "new users who lack the accumulated knowledge of experienced consumers." it is a great starting point.

https://greencamp.com/marijuana-terms/

Ganjaprenuer
Besides liking the term (who thinks of these word mash-ups anyway?) I like the fact that Ganjapreneur brings you a long list of ma-

rijuana **slang**. Each word is hyperlinked to its own page. Unlike the other sources in this list, Ganjaprenuer focuses on slang. Like Colorado Pot Guide, each term includes its use in a sentence. In addition, Ganjapreneur gives your related terms at the bottom of the page. Plus each page has unrelated public domain old photos for each definition which made me scratch my head wondering how much the authors smoked while creating the pages.

https://www.ganjapreneur.com/marijuana-slang/

Westword

Finally, Westword has a blog article called, "Dispensary Dictionary: Cannabis Definitions for Rookies" by Scott Lentz. This is a great page to be familiar with as clients who frequent dispensaries will probably use these terms.

https://www.westword.com/marijuana/dispensary-dictionary-cannabis-definitions-for-rookies-9626635

Apps for your Phone

The Marijuana Handbook

Available in the Lite (free) and paid (42.99) versions in the itunes store and available on Amazon for the kindle. It is currently not available for android. Last updated in 2016

https://www.amazon.com/Fallacy-Studios-Marijuana-Handbook/dp/B007PTW1SI

https://itunes.apple.com/us/app/marijuana-handbook/id470296810

https://itunes.apple.com/us/app/marijuana-handbook-lite/id477750914

Marijuana Dictionary A-Z

Free. It is available on both android and apple platforms. Last updated in 2016.

With 380 definitions, the Marijuana Dictionary A-Z has some great information for beginners.

https://play.google.com/store/apps/details?id=com.prestigeworldwid.mjdictionary

https://itunes.apple.com/au/app/marijuana-dictionary-a-z/id1082228425

CANNABIS CONSUMPTION CALCULATOR (CCC)

Overview

The CCC is a one page information gathering tool to

You can download it here: http://bit.ly/cannabiscalculator

Instructions For Administering

History
There are many forms for cannabis and the list seems to be growing regularly. This tool groups products into 5 categories. It does not include products used primarily in medical (versus recreational) uses (such as transdermal patches and suppositories).

Lifetime / Last 30 Days: Enter a Yes / No response.

Flower
If the client does not know, use 15% for the THC

How much have you smoked: it may be difficult for a client to think in terms of gram weight. They might be better able to think in terms of "joints" – even though that is imprecise depending on who rolled it, paper etc. It is our most current best measurement that most can picture. Fractions are acceptable (e.g., "1/3 of joint")

Shared: unlike other products, Flowers are complicated because multiple people might be sharing. When calculating milligrams consumed for an individual, will to divide what was consumed by the number of people sharing.

Calculations: Show your math. Don't calculate this in your head. First, convert THC percent to milligrams, simply move the decimal point over. 20% THC = 200 milligrams THC per gram.

Then estimate the serving by how much flower was smoked. A half gram of dry flower is a common amount found in most joints. So if a client reports smoking half a joint that means a quarter (1/4) gram of dry flower.

Next divide that number by the number of people sharing. So if two people were sharing and smoked half a joint, the individual consumption would be one eighth (1/8) of a gram.

Multiplying milligrams THC per gram with the amount of grams consumed provide you with the highest potential serving.

However smoking flower is an inefficient method for taking THC – much of the THC is lost in the sidestream when smoking – up to 70% in some estimates. You will also want to factor in lost THC. Smoking We will factor in a 50% loss to calculate probable serving.

So to calculate serving, multiply milligrams THC per gram by the amount consumed by the THC loss.

In the preceding example that would be

> 200 milligrams THC per gram x 1/8 gram x 50% = 12.5 milligrams

Example:
A client reports smoking a joint every day which he shares with two roommates and THC is 22%.

That means 220 milligrams of THC per gram which means 110 milligrams in a half gram joint which means 36 milligrams shared per joint as the potential serving . Assuming a 50% loss from smoking means a probable serving of 18 milligrams.

Vape
Most prefilled vape pens shut off after a period of inhaling. For example a pen might deliver a 2 mg potential serving from one 7 second inhale. Therefore a partial inhale of 3 seconds should deliver a 1 mg probable serving.

Concentrates
Clearly labeled, dosing should be easily calculated.

Edibles
Also clearly labeled and often packaged in individual servings (e.g., lozenges) or easily divided (e.g., chocolate bar).

Have you ever overdone it: avoiding the word overdose, ask if the person has felt like they took too many edibles at one time and got "too high" or "too wasted". You are assessing the degree they are mood seeking or chasing the high.

Infused Oils
These should be the easiest to calculate as the THC per drop is pretty clear (typically 1 milligram).

Microdosing. You are looking for repeatedly trying to be a little high all day long.

HOOKLES

"If you can't measure something, you can't understand it. If you can't understand it, you can't control it."

H. JAMES HARRINGTON

What We Need For Marijuana And Marijuana Is A Hookle.

At the liquor store, liquor bottles have a number on the label designating proof. At the grocery store, packaged products have a number on the label designating calories. At the marijuana store, products need a number on the label designating amount of THC. A hookle is a made up term I made up to illustrate a system of measurement for THC.

Now, I fully understand that smoking get's you high faster than sublingual absorption which is faster than digestion. I want you to put the method of consumption to the side for a moment as we fast forward to a time where THC is labeled in hookles.

In this hypothetical illustration, let's say consuming 2 hookles left the average person feeling relaxed for two hours and that 4 hookles impacted their motor skills (they definitely shouldn't be driving after consuming 4 hookles) and at 6 hookles the average person hallucinated and at 8 hookles they fell asleep.

Just imagine.

Imagine, when you browsed through the assortment of products in the marijuana store, everything was clearly labeled with hookles and serving size in big, bold, easy-to-read numbers.

Consumers could easily navigate products and start off with a serving size of 1 hookle with a full awareness of the impact of more than one hookles consumed in quick succession.

On top of that consumers knew how hookles were metabolized for effect for the average person. If you smoked one hookle you would feel the effects within three minutes. If you absorbed a hookle under your tongue you would feel the effects within fifteen minutes. If you ate a hookle you would feel the effects within forty-five minutes.

Equipped with this information about hookles, the average person could plan out their evening recreational consumption.

And just like people metabolize alcohol differently based on size, history and more, we would learn the same about ourselves with how we metabolize hookles.

People might 'say things like, "You haven't smoked marijuana in a long time, you shouldn't have more than 1 hookle." Or, "I'm a big guy and have smoked for a while, I can handle my hookles." And even a spouse might suggest, "Honey, you have had one too many hookles, I think I should drive -- you smoked 2 hookles and just ate 2 more which won't hit you for 45 minutes when we are driving home and you will have 4 hookles in your system which is dangerous for driving."

Doctors and public health professionals could educate the public about the adverse effects of too many hookles. They could even make recommendations of how many hookles per day or week are healthy and how many are not, just like they do with alcohol today.

You might even read in the newspaper about some study from France that concludes consuming one hookle each night before bed is associated with decrease risk of heart attack. And recommending a hookle before bed becomes a standard recommendation of medical professionals across the nation for people with high blood pressure.

Until 3 years after that when another study comes out that shows no relationship between hookle consumption and heart attacks.

None of this. Not the informed choices at the marijuana store. Not the conversation with your spouse as you ponder getting behind the wheel of a car. Not the education from medical professionals. Not the conflicting studies by researches. None of this can take place until we have a concept in place like the hookle.

BIBLIOGRAPHY: A CURATED READING LIST

I tapped into hundreds of sources in researching the topic. Here are my favorite resources for further learning. There's a lot of information so I have attempted to help you out with a rating and overview for each article, paper and source.

Must Reads

Marijuana vs. Alcohol: Which Is Really Worse for Your Health?
https://www.livescience.com/42738-marijuana-vs-alcohol-health-effects.html

> Rating: ****
> Overview: Includes short and long term consequences of marijuana and alcohol use.
> What I like about this page: Although written in 2014, much of the information is applicable; presentation appears bias-free; quick read.

Marijuana Equivalency in Portion and Dosage
https://www.colorado.gov/pacific/sites/default/files/MED%20Equivalency_Final%2008102015.pdf

> Rating: *****

Overview: Comparative study by the Colorado Department of Revenue, including a section on pharmacological equivalencies.
What I like about this pdf: While written from an economics perspective primarily, there is much that health professionals can learn regarding the diversity of marijuana products and how their potency compares.

Variation in cannabis potency and prices in a newly legal market: evidence from 30 million cannabis sales in Washington state
https://www.ncbi.nlm.nih.gov/pubmed/28556310

Rating: ****
Overview: Brief summary with link to the 45-page article that you can read for free.
What I like about this pdf: The shift from cannabis flower to other marijuana products is apparent from this large study.

Mythbusters: Cannabis potency
https://www.drugfoundation.org.nz/matters-of-substance/november-2010/cannabis-potency/

Rating: *****
Overview: Short article from New Zealand that explores the fear-tactic hype from some health professionals.
What I like about this page: Summed up in the last sentence: "Perhaps we should really be asking, 'Are cannabis users getting higher or are they using less cannabis to achieve the same effects?'"

How To Dose Cannabis In Its Various Forms
https://www.royalqueenseeds.com/blog-how-to-dose-cannabis-in-its-various-forms-n1013

Rating: ***
Overview: One-page overview of marijuana products.
What I like about this page: Nice introduction, although I think the dosages identified are rather high (5-10 mg for microdosing seems rather high – unless a gram in Great Brit-

ain is different than a gram in the United States)

Edibles Dosing Chart: Interpreting Potency in Infused Cannabis Products
https://www.leafly.com/news/cannabis-101/cannabis-edibles-dosage-guide-chart

> Rating: *****
> Overview: Easy to understand chart you can print out for your office.
> What I like about this page: This chart seems to have a more reasonable measurement of THC than the website above (from Royal Queen Seeds). I would print it out, laminate it and use it as a guide for sorting through myriad of consumption options.

What's Hot in the Edibles Market
https://www.cannabisbusinesstimes.com/article/spotlight-whats-hot-in-the-us-edibles-market/

> Rating: *****
> Overview: Written in 2018, a projection of what we might see in the next 5 years.
> What I like about this page: I love the pie chart showing the projected breakdown of edibles in 2022, driven my small amounts of THC for low dosing.

How To Combat Cannabis-Caused Anxiety
https://www.royalqueenseeds.com/blog-how-to-combat-cannabis-caused-anxiety-n664

> Rating: **
> Overview: A short and somewhat inaccurate article but a good primer to get health professionals thinking. (The article instructs the reader to "try to eat or drink something. It will have an instant impact on the chemicals in your bloodstream." Instant impact? Well, that is ridiculous).
> What I like about this page: I included this article because I think counselors in the future will need to know how to do

marijuana psychological first aid

Bud Digest
https://buddigest.com

> Rating: ***
> Overview: Marijuana news
> What I like about this page: Seems to a up to date news feed about marijuana in the news.

General Information

DrugFacts - Marijuana National Institute of Drug Abuse (USA)
https://d14rmgtrwzf5a.cloudfront.net/sites/default/files/drugfacts-marijuana.pdf

> Rating: *
> Overview: 9-page "fact sheet" written by the National institute on Drug Abuse.
> What I like about this pdf: It is a good primer, although biased as it focused on the consequences of extreme heavy marijuana use and not any benefits.

Cannabis Parent Update from the Community Prevention Initiative (CPI)
Funded through the California Department of Health Care Services (DHCS), Substance Use Disorder Program, Policy and Fiscal Division (SUD-PPFD) with training and technical assistance (TTA) administered through the Center for Applied Research Solutions (CARS).

http://www.ca-cpi.org/docs/Cannabis-Parent-Update-Brochure.pdf

> Rating: ***
> Overview: Short brochure-style with brief information from the state of California.
> What I like about this pdf: Written for parents with a focus on prevention, a good orientation to marijuana with only a few key facts to digest; you won't get overloaded with infor-

mation.

Black Market

Cannabis Black Market Thriving Despite Legalization
https://www.forbes.com/sites/nickkovacevich/2019/03/13/cannabis-black-market-thriving-despite-legalization/#76f3bfe75ea2

> Rating: ****
> Overview: March 2019 article about black markets in areas where marijuana is legal.
> What I like about this page: Clearly points out the drivers of continuing black market – "local opposition, high taxes and onerous regulations." Once these come in line, the black markets will go away.

Marijuana Legalization Makes Black Market Better In Prohibition States
https://www.forbes.com/sites/mikeadams/2018/11/13/marijuana-legalization-makes-black-market-better-in-prohibition-states/#5f2078aa2633

> Rating: *****
> Overview: 2018 article written from a political, social and economic perspective.
> What I like about this page: Cannabis edibles are on the rise in the black market too!

Despite Legalization, Marijuana Black Market Hides In Plain Sight
https://www.npr.org/2018/05/16/610579599/despite-legalization-marijuana-black-market-hides-in-plain-sight

> Rating: ****
> Overview: Short read about the continuing of a black market with legalization.
> What I like about this page: Clearly identifies the economic drivers of a black market. Did you ever see the movie, "Smokey and the Bandit"? While not entirely accurate in its premise about Coors beer being legal in certain parts of

the country, at the time of the movie, Coors beer was only available in certain parts of the country (the western US) and there was a thriving market for Coors beer sold person to person in other parts of the country (the eastern US).

Business & Regulation

Business Readiness Guidebook for OLCC Marijuana Operations
https://www.oregon.gov/olcc/marijuana/Documents/BusinessReadinessGuide_RecreationalMarijuana.pdf

>Rating: ****
>Overview: From the state or Oregon, a business primer for the marijuana entrepreneur.
>What I like about this pdf: Highly detailed read about running a legal marijuana business – a good overview of the regulations that the marijuana industry must abide by.

Decarboxylation

What Is Decarboxylation, and Why Does Your Cannabis Need It?
https://www.leafly.com/news/cannabis-101/what-is-decarboxylation

>Rating: ***
>Overview: An interesting article (and added expense for the home grower)
>What I like about this page: Really shows how the home grower has a lot to consider when producing their own marijuana flower to smoke. Also shows the maturing of the marijuana hobby market.

Dosing

Cannabis Dosing Guide - Project CBD
https://www.projectcbd.org/sites/projectcbd/files/downloads/projectcbd_cannabis-dosing-guide_brochure.pdf

>Rating: *
>Overview: Short, brochure-format about using marijuana written from a cannabis-is-medicine perspective.

What I like about this pdf: Clearly shows the hype that the legal marijuana proponents / industry are putting out there. "Personalized *Medicine*"?! You can't get any more hyped than that!

Sample Dosing Guidelines – Tilray
https://www.tilray.ca/media/magefan_blog/Tilray_Sample_Dosing_Guidelines_03.pdf

Rating: ***
Overview: Straightforward brochure about marijuana servings.
What I like about this pdf: Very little hype from the marijuana industry. Although it does repeat the mantra, "Start low, go slow", Tilray does acknowledge that, "currently there and no established uniform dosing schedules."

Practical considerations in medical cannabis administration and dosing
http://www.cpsa.ca/wp-content/uploads/2018/08/MacCallum-Russo-Practical-Considerations-in-Medical-Cannabis-Administrat....pdf

Rating: *****
Overview: Detailed information about dosing from the European Journal of Internal Medicine.
What I like about this pdf: You may need to read it two or three times to fully understand and retain the information presented but it is hype-free and pragmatic in its application.

Clinical Guidance: for the use of medicinal cannabis products in Queensland - August 2018
https://www.health.qld.gov.au/__data/assets/pdf_file/0023/634163/med-cannabis-clinical-guide.pdf

Rating: ***
Overview: From New Zealand, this article identifies dosing and legal requirements for New Zealand

What I like about this pdf: While still echoing the mantra put out by the marijuana industry (start low go slow), there are some valuable references in the Appendix worth checking out.

A Review of Medical Cannabis Studies relating to Chemical Compositions and Dosages for Qualifying Medical Conditions - May 2018
Minnesota Department of Health

https://health.state.mn.us/people/cannabis/docs/practitioners/dosagesandcompositions2018.pdf

Rating: *****
Overview: From the state of Minnesota, an 81-page document on medical conditions appropriate for marijuana usage and their respective dosage.
What I like about this pdf: Long and difficult read at times but well worth it for health professionals looking for an unbiased perspective on medical marijuana, this study of the studies is an invaluable resource and reference.

Cannabis Dosage Guide: How to Accurately Measure THC Levels
https://ardentcannabis.com/accurately-dose-cannabis/

Rating: *****
Overview: Overview of measuring THC levels and converting these to grams
What I like about this page: Home test kits! This really shows the growth of this industry. Plus converting THC to grams instructions.

How to Calculate THC Dosages in Cannabis Edibles
https://www.royalqueenseeds.com/blog-how-to-calculate-thc-dosages-in-cannabis-edibles-n238

Rating: ***
Overview: From Royal Queen Seeds a clear guide to cooking with cannabis and determining how much THV to put in your culinary creations.

What I like about this page: Straightforward conversion advice, though, like the previous reference from Royal Queen Seeds, the numbers don't seem to sync with US calculations (see article by Ardent Cannabis, above).

The THC Dosage Guide: Flower, Edibles, Concentrates and More
https://keytocannabis.com/blogs/cannabis/the-thc-dosage-guide-flower-edibles-concentrates-and-more

Rating: ****
Overview: Quick survey of product types and guidelines.
What I like about this page: I like the pictures of flower and weights. It is a nice orientation for the new user and clarification for the experienced user.

DSM 5

A Guide to DSM 5 Criteria for Substance Use Disorders
https://www.verywellmind.com/dsm-5-criteria-for-substance-use-disorders-21926

Rating: ***
Overview: Brief overview of the 11 criteria for a substance use disorder diagnosis as outlined in the DSM-5
What I like about this page: Well written, and includes information on severity specifiers.

Cannabis Use Disorder or Problematic Marijuana Use
https://www.verywellmind.com/cannabis-use-disorder-22295

Rating: ***
Overview: Brief orientation to the DSM-5 diagnosis.
What I like about this page: Articulates the shift from dependence in the DSM-4 to the disorder (with specifiers) in the DSM-5

Cannabis Use Disorder DSM-5, 305.20, 304.30
https://www.theravive.com/therapedia/cannabis-use-disorder-dsm--5%2C-305.20%2C-304.30

Rating: ***

Overview: Outlines specific considerations in making a diagnosis of Cannabis Use Disorder

What I like about this page: Includes risk factors, differential diagnosis and comorbidity factors.

Edibles

Four Ways Edibles Can Hit You Faster
https://www.leafly.com/news/strains-products/fast-acting-edibles

Rating: ***

Overview: Information from Leafy – the website for connecting to dispensaries and learning more about marijuana.

What I like about this page: It is noteworthy in the medical / dosing context to see this article that is at its core about how to get higher faster from marijuana.

5 Tips to Safely Dose and Enjoy Cannabis Edibles
https://www.leafly.com/news/cannabis-101/5-tips-to-safely-dose-and-enjoy-cannabis-edibles

Rating: ***

Overview: Simple one-page guide to not over-consuming edibles.

What I like about this page: "We are past the days of playing Russian roulette to determine edible doses." Nicely said. And nice guidance to consider what is in your stomach, tolerance while being patient.

Cannabis edibles: 5 potent tips to make your experience more enjoyable
https://www.straight.com/cannabis/995326/cannabis-edibles-5-potent-tips-make-your-experience-more-enjoyable

Rating: **

Overview: Written from the pro-legalization perspective, introduces the "entourage" effect

What I like about this page: Interesting to see the hype from the author who pronounces herself as a fitness enthusiast concerned about "eating clean and eliminating sugar and artificial additives" while promoting marijuana edibles.

The Beginner's Guide to Edibles
https://lifehacker.com/the-beginners-guide-to-edibles-1821047006

> Rating: ***
> Overview: Short, introductory article from the folks at lifehacker.
> What I like about this page: Simple and to the point, not a lot of hype. A good read if you are thinking of trying edibles out.

Weed & Marijuana Edibles: How To Dose & Ingest Properly
https://weedmaps.com/learn/products-and-how-to-consume/edibles/

> Rating: ***
> Overview: Overview of edibles including how they work and how they are made.
> What I like about this page: Nice pictures and recommended servicing sizes, though the serving size for the new-to-marijuana user seems particularly high.

Marijuana 101: Calculating how much THC is in your homemade edibles
https://www.thegrowthop.com/cannabis-culture/marijuana-101-calculating-how-much-thc-is-in-your-homemade-edibles

> Rating: *
> Overview: Very short article about cooking with marijuana
> What I like about this page: The information on potency (grams) is helpful in understanding how the THC in marijuana flower is related to the THC in edibles.

Medical Use

Cannabis or Excedrin for Migraines – How They Compare

https://cannabismd.com/health/headaches/marijuana-or-excedrin-for-migraines-how-they-compare/

> Rating: ***
> Overview: More of an editorial than a report on a research study comparing Excedrin and marijuana.
> What I like about this page: This is the future. Today: Excedrin (Acetaminophen 250 mg, Aspirin 250 mg, and Caffeine 65 mg.) Five year from now: Cool-name-for-marketing-purposes (Acetaminophen 250 mg, Aspirin 250 mg, and THC 5 g.)

Microdosing

I Microdosed Weed For a Week. Here's What Happened
https://www.cosmopolitan.com/lifestyle/a19862479/microdosing-cannabis-for-a-week/

> Rating: *****
> Overview: Lengthy blog post about one person's experience with sustained microdosing.
> What I like about this page: Living life kind-of high – but not really high; microdosing is a potential slippery slope for those prone to addiction. A great, honest, week-long memoir and good orientation for health professionals to this behavior.

Microdosing With Cannabis: Benefits Without the Buzz
https://www.leafly.com/news/cannabis-101/microdosing-weed-guide

> Rating: **
> Overview: Article about microdosing but not consuming to the point where you feel even a little high.
> What I like about this page: An alternative use of the word microdosing that health professionals should be familiar with (as opposed to microdosing to feel a-little-high-but-not-wasted, though hype-filled with statements like "Microdosing is something that is very personal."

The Essential Guide to Microdosing Marijuana
https://thethirdwave.co/microdosing/marijuana/

> Rating: **
> Overview: Held out at *the* step-by-step guide and written from a marijuana-can-cure everything perspective.
> What I like about this page: Lots of references for those exploring the subject. Plus this quote which is a great reflection of the pro-marijuana medicalized mumbo jumbo that is out there: "A microdose is relative to the threshold dose of a psychedelic—that is, the lowest dose of the drug that creates a perceptible effect—and therefore it is below that threshold, resulting in a sub-perceptual effect that is subtle without markedly influencing your mood or mindset." Gee whiz.

Patches

Cannabis Patches For Pain Relief
https://www.royalqueenseeds.com/blog-cannabis-patches-for-pain-relief-n708

> Rating: ***
> Overview: Introductory article about marijuana patches
> What I like about this page: It is good to be familiar with the various forms of marijuana consumption.

Potency

Is Cannabis Really More Potent Today Than It Was 20 Years Ago?
https://www.originscannabis.com/marijuana-potency/

> Rating: ***
> Overview: Short history of the increase in potency
> What I like about this page: While written from a clear bias toward marijuana, this article does throw some cold water on the scare tactics that some health professionals fan the flames of.

Propaganda

The Truth About Marijuana booklet

https://www.drugfreeworld.org/sites/default/files/truth-about-marijuana-booklet-en.pdf

> Rating: ***
> Overview: Anytime you read the word "truth" in a title you know you are in for some propaganda and the Foundation for a Drug-Free World does not disappoint in this pdf.
> What I like about this pdf: Nothing. Except it is scary that some people swallow this hook line and sinker.

Terminology

Weed Guide: A Visual Glossary of Cannabis Terminology
https://keytocannabis.com/blogs/cannabis/photos-weed-glossary-common-cannabis-terminology

> Rating: *****
> Overview: Short glossary of terms with graphics and photos.
> What I like about this page: Lots of pictures! Good orientation for people who may be unfamiliar with every aspect of marijuana, the industry and products.

THC / THCA / THC Levels / CBD

How to Assess THC and CBD Levels in Cannabis Strains and Products
https://www.leafly.com/news/science-tech/how-to-assess-thc-cbd-levels-in-cannabis-strains-products

> Rating: ****
> Overview: THC, THC-A, decarboxylation, formulas and more.
> What I like about this page: A lot of information in a little bit of space. You might need to review this article a few times but being familiar with these terms will help you navigate conversations with your patients / clients.

What is THC?
https://www.royalqueenseeds.com/blog-what-is-thc-n70

Rating: *****
Overview: Short blog post about tetrahydrocannabinol, is the chemical that causes the psychological effects of marijuana

What I like about this page: Great graphics, photos and information from the pro-marijuana folks at Royal Queen Seeds.

The Difference Between CBD Oil and Cannabis Oil
https://www.royalqueenseeds.com/blog-the-difference-between-cbd-oil-and-cannabis-oil-n616

Rating: **
Overview: Brief marketing-shaded overview about products in Europe.

What I like about this page: Worth a quick glance if only to appreciate the every diversifying marijuana industry. It reminds me of all the different iterations of Coca-Cola (Coca-Cola, Diet Coke, Coke Zero Sugar, Cherry Coke, Vanilla Coke, etc., etc., etc. I say be prepared for Coke THC, Coke CBD, Coke THC/CBD 1:1 and more in the future!).

THCA and THC: What's the Difference?
https://weedmaps.com/learn/cannabis-and-your-body/difference-between-thca-thc/

Rating: **
Overview: Brief introduction with a nice graphic – and a reminder to know what decarboxylation is.

What I like about this page: As a health professional you will need to know this at some point in the very near future and this is a great introduction.

Vaping

Everything You Need to Know About Pre-Filled Oil Vape Cartridges
https://www.leafly.com/news/strains-products/what-are-pre-filled-cannabis-oil-vape-cartridges

Rating: *****

Overview: Detailed article about vaping.
What I like about this page: Really is everything you need to know. Great resource for health professionals to educate themselves as well as in their efforts to educate consumers.

A Beginner's Guide to Vaping Cannabis: Where to Start
http://www.maximumyield.com/a-beginners-guide-to-vaping-cannabis-where-to-start/2/4677

Rating: ***
Overview: Brief article about vaping directed at first time buyers
What I like about this page: Information light with links to other articles on the site if you want to go deeper into a topic.

How vape pens allow you to better manage your high
https://mashable.com/article/everything-to-know-about-vape-weed-pens-tech/

Rating: ***
Overview: XX
What I like about this page: This is one of the reasons we will see less traditional smoking of marijuana – it is not just that products like edibles and vaping are easier to use and less noticeable – it is that they (tinctures and vaping in particular) allow for greater control and management of your high.

How to Use a Vape Pen
https://my420tours.com/how-to-use-a-vape-pen/

Rating: ***
Overview: Brief article on vape pens.
What I like about this page: Some great graphics – almost infographic in nature – and organized in a list format (e.g., 5 ways to XYZ).

END NOTES

[i] https://www.denverpost.com/2018/05/09/marijuana-cannabis-pregnancy-nausea-colorado-study/

[ii] https://www.newsweek.com/man-who-ate-marijuana-lollipop-had-heart-attack-caused-fearful-hallucinations-1324067

[iii] https://www.cbsnews.com/news/georgia-teen-dies-from-drinking-too-much-water-gatorade/)

[iv] https://www.ncbi.nlm.nih.gov/pmc/articles/PMC3615510

[v] https://www.fireengineering.com/articles/print/volume-165/issue-11/departments/fireems/bath-salts-and-synthetic-marijuana-an-emerging-threat.html

[vi] https://www.originscannabis.com/marijuana-potency

[vii] https://www.zdnet.com/article/marijuana-means-business-everything-you-need-to-know-about-the-cannabis-industry/

[viii] https://www.cnbc.com/2018/06/28/from-sleep-aids-to-beverages-the-future-of-cannabis-is-in-products-c.html

[ix] https://www.cannabisbusinesstimes.com/article/spotlight-whats-hot-in-the-us-edibles-market/

[x] https://www.leafly.com/news/cannabis-101/costs-of-cannabis-growing-vs-buying

[xi] https://www.theatlantic.com/health/archive/2019/02/weed-active-ingredients-yeast/583765

[xii] https://www.outsideonline.com/2390779/cannabis-beer

[xiii] Wikipedia, https://en.wikipedia.org/wiki/Cannabis

[xiv] https://www.reformer.com/stories/retired-bf-woman-completes-long-trail,305638

LIST OF CONTRIBUTORS

Robin Rieske
Robin Rieske has been a Certified Prevention Consultant, advocate and community organizer in Vermont for over 27 years. She enjoys hiking, dancing and sharing time with friends and family.

Susan M. Williams
Susan Williams is a Licensed Alcohol and Drug Counselor who has been working in the addictions field since 1993. She has worked with clients of the Department of Corrections and Project CRASH. She teaches "Tai Chi for Fall Prevention" in Bellows Falls, VT, and enjoys hiking (she is a Long Trail end-to-ender[xiv]), gardening, cooking, and vipassana meditation.

ABOUT SCOTT GRAHAM

Scott is a business and career coach from Boston, MA. When he is not coaching people to be their best, he participates in Tough Mudders, hikes, works on a farm, practices Vipassana meditation, or volunteers as an EMT and firefighter.

OTHER BOOKS BY SCOTT GRAHAM

Ten Things You Need to Know About Coaching Before You Get a Coach

Motivational Interviewing Made Easy

Work Exchange: A Handbook for Hosts

How to Become More Linkable… …and Likeable on LinkedIn

Check! Your Guide to Creating a Life Transforming Bucket List

Growing & Using Good King Henry

Make Time Your Superhero Power!

Get Off Your Ass & Mow The Grass!

CONTACT SCOTT GRAHAM

True Azimuth, LLC
265 Franklin Street
Suite 1702
Boston, MA 02110

Phone: (617) 475-0081

Website: http://TrueAzimuth.biz
Email: sgraham@TrueAzimuth.biz
Skype: TrueAzimuth
Twitter: @TrueAzimuth
Facebook: http://www.facebook.com/trueazimuthcoaching
Google+: http://plus.google.com/+TrueazimuthBiz-BusinessCoach
LinkedIn: http://www.linkedin.com/company/true-azimuth-llc